VERTIGO – call of the void

VERTIGO – call of the void

by

Wolfgang H. Zangemeister

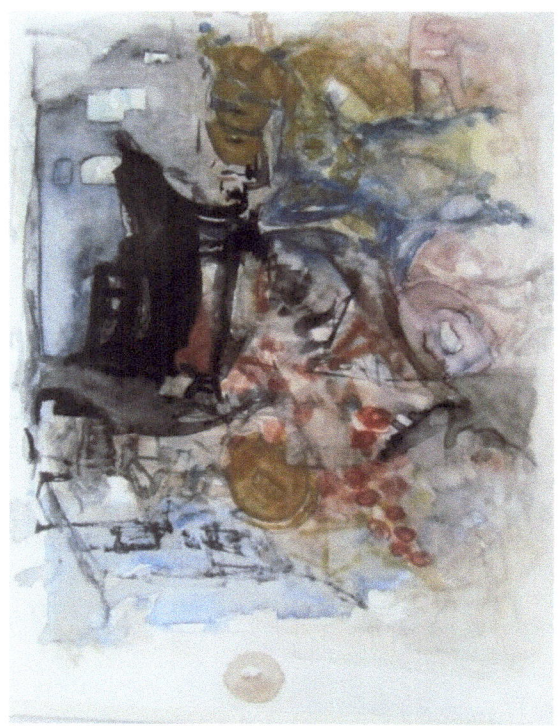

Hamburg 2020

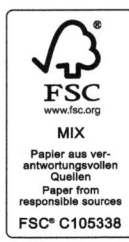

Bibliografische Information der Deutschen Nationalbibliothek:
Die Deutsche Nationalbibliothek verzeichnet diese Publikation in der Deutschen Nationalbibliografie;
detaillierte bibliografische Daten sind im Internet über
http://dnb.d-nb.de abrufbar.

© 2020 Wolfgang H. Zangemeister
Satz, Herstellung und Verlag: BoD- Books on Demand, Norderstedt
ISBN: 978-3-7519-8670-0

Content

Imbalance and destabilization of space orientation   9

Borderline between two perceptual settings   11

Mixed emotions and Anxiety   14

Time course of dizziness   14

Dizziness – Functional Anatomy   16

Systematic and Time-defined Vertigo   17

Dizziness in a stricter sense   17

Clinical analysis of the ambiguous vertigo information   18

Vertigo – the most common type of dizziness:
Frequent Diagnoses   19

Diagnostic Tests   21

Dizziness of psychosomatic origin   22

Psychosomatic and Psychogenic   25

Phobic Vertigo   26

Phobia and Psychoanalysis   28

Fearful Dreams   28

Incomprehensible and confusing emotions   29

Regression: Fear and Psychogenic Vertigo   30

Vertigo is not a disease entity but a multifaceted, unspecific symptom. More than 300 diseases might trigger dizziness. So, in the diagnosis of vertigo disorders the doctor is bound to have a very broad spectrum of associations of likely causes of this symptom. The ethymology of the term *vertigo* has a wide range of meanings. Vertigo is the most common type of dizziness. Dizziness comes from dwindling (Old High German: *swintan*) which means to lessen. Such a physical process would be addressed as consumptive. In the days of Sturm und Drang (*storm and stress*) vertigo changes to the dizziness of trembling, triggered by strong sensations, an emotional experience: You get dizzy, perhaps unconscious. In English, "*to swindle*" means to cheat. This meaning was adopted by the German-speaking countries and used in the German-Dutch business practices to secure an exchange here with an even bigger there: The proposal is therefore synonymous with the concept of Cross Riding, i.e. *Wechselreiterei*. The original noun from the Latin word vertigo from *vertere,* turn around, rotate, was expressed as *swintilot* in old high German and later replaced by *swindel* in Middle High German. If we follow the Latin word vertigo into English of our time, we find two distinct definitions. One was used by Lord Brain[1]: *Vertigo is a state of disordered orientation regarding the body and space.* This reflects the common parlance. By contrast, the Dutch ENT doctor Jongkees[2] defined vertigo as: The sensation of movement – i.e. a designation emphasizing the vestibular character of dizziness. On the other hand, the term dizziness accounts for short-term disruption of the relationship of the individual subject within space. The original meaning of dizzy was: Foolish, mentally insteady, whirling with mad rapidity, stupid, silly – psychologically insecure and wheeling with crazy speed. This certainly contains psychological components of its ambivalent meaning.

In the late eighteenth century "vertigo" concerned medical anthropology, the subject of which was the spiritual life of man. At that time, this still concerned philosophy, while the approach was empirical and oriented towards the observational practices of natural science. Man in his combination of body and mind became the object of observation. Their pathological deviations were intended to provide information about the nature of man. Vertigo was one of the phenomena that were clearly localized at the border between body and soul. The Jewish physician and philosopher Marcus Herz [3], a student of Immanuel Kant, described and classified the phenomena that led to vertigo and dizziness: "an illness of the soul – independent of its physical or mental causes". Behind this was a sensualist theory of the life of the soul, which was based on the basic ability of the soul to have conceptions that followed a certain rhythm: our conceptions can only be clear and distinct if they follow each other at an appropriate time interval. This meant that the inner conceptions must have a suitable "healthy" speed; for if the successive conceptions are too fast, then dizziness and vertigo arise.

When the neurologists of the 19th century dealt with the phenomenon of vertigo, they did this assuming that a more detailed analysis could improve the knowledge of the vestibular organs, that is of the vestibular system, and provide important information on the structure and function of the brain. For Purkinje[4], who undertook self-tests by quickly turning around his body axis with open eyes, dizziness was the general feeling that is in your mind such as fear in your chest.

Imbalance and destabilization of space orientation

After the discovery of the labyrinth in the inner ear as origin of vestibular vertigo, dizziness became increasingly understood as a physical injury symptom. Today's definition of vertigo surpasses the question if vertigo is an objective disturbance of balance or a subjective illusion. Dizziness is now defined as a state of a more or less abrupt onset of imbalance, associated with vegetative and painful symptoms, while feeling a strong disturbance of body-space relationship. In 1966, H. Stenger[5] defined dizziness as a disorientation in space, which is accompanied by signs of the neuro-vegetative system and unpleasant emotions. This has to be distinguished from a non-directional imbalance, which is primarily a failure of the postural and movement coordination. Less systematic, vestibular vertigo i.e. vertigo in the strict sense, is an impairment of consciousness and postural motor functions with disappearance of sense.

Already Hippocrates has described vertigo as a cerebral syndrome: skoto´dinos or vertigo tenebricosa. Imbalance of sensory systems of reference – eye, labyrinth, somatosensory system – already physiologically leads to dizziness due to this "mismatch". Pathological vertigo also arises from a conflict, a dysequilibrium. Failures of the vestibular system, of its connections to the cerebellum, double vision as a result of sudden eye muscle paralysis, or body position and movement disturbances caused by disorders of peripheral nerve or spinal tracts: all lead to dysequilibrium. In all cases there is an imbalance, a destabilization of space orientation and dizziness. In early experiments by Paul Vogel and Paul Kestenbaum[6] from the thirties concerning optokinetic vertigo, the test subject was asked to stand under an optical rotary wheel, where the interior was papered with white and black stripes, and a small mark had to be fixated. They were able to show that with concentration onto the irritating rotation stimulus, next to a subjectively noted dizziness, unsteadiness and falling tendency of the subject, adjustment operations were generated with change of posture. These could not be determined by the subject itself, only by an observer. In addition, with an identical stimulus exposure, depending on the inner attitude of the subject a subjective apparent movement was generated and not just vertigo. Both settings cannot be simultaneously sensed and thought. A phenomenon that is reminiscent of the perception of ambiguous images that cannot be perceived and thought at the same time in their ambiguity. Additionally, there is the transition from one setting to the other within a moment of emptiness; this is reported by the subject only, but not by the investigator, who cannot perceive a postural change.

Borderline between two perceptual settings

Dizziness occurs not only in response to an irritating stimulus. It also marks the borderline between two perceptual settings. Because of the frequent discrepancy of vertigo as a subjective phenomenon and objectively relevant examination findings, the symptom *vertigo* bears initially a limited value in terms of the location of a certain vertigo-inducing disorder. However, via a rational analysis of the subjectively accompanying symptoms and signs – like e.g. emesis and double vision – one could infer functional anatomical background. Among unselected patients vertigo is one of the most common complaints.

Dizziness affects approximately 20%-40% of people at some point in time while about 7.5%-10% have vertigo. About 5% have vertigo in a given year. It becomes more common with age and affects women two to three times more often than men. Vertigo accounts for about 2-3% of emergency department visits in the developed world.

Patients from general practices in 65% claim to have suffered in the previous 12 months from dizziness, 18% even reported about frequent vertigo. In a survey of 30 000 people in Baden-Württemberg, 20% of men and 40% of women claimed to suffer occasionally from vertigo. Of 16 000 patients of the German Diagnostic Clinic at least 19% reported dizzy states. In addition, complaints about vertigo are particularly frequent as accompanying symptom of neurotic disorders. Patients with anxiety disorders reported in 78% vertigo. Among the patients of the Neurological Clinic of Hamburg University (1990 – 2011) who did not show an organic disease and where a primary psychiatric disorder had been postulated, dizziness was the second frequent complaint after headaches.

Further analysis with mapping to different types of vertigo leads to vertigo as a symptom. Under 50 years of age the frequency of dizziness is prevalent in 40% of large unselected patient groups below 50 years – over 50 years it increases to about 70%.

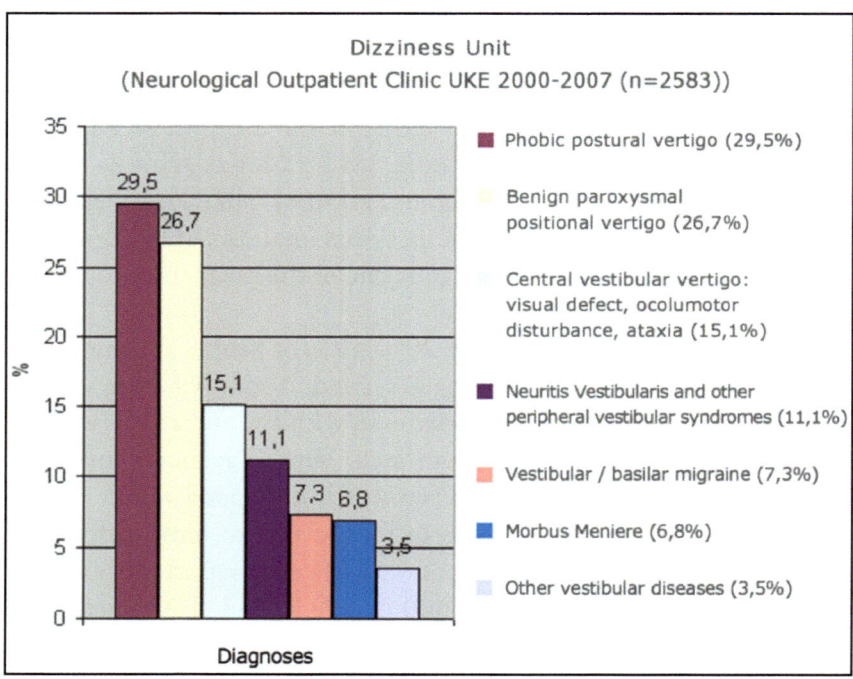

Fig.1. *Overview of the years 2000 – 2007 from the Dizziness Unit of the Neurology Clinic at the University Hospital Hamburg UKE.*

At old age, dizziness and unsteadiness are often seen as "normal" part of aging. That this is incorrect, and is demonstrated by a variety of studies in this area. Doctor Klaus Jahn[7] and coauthors recently reported in a comprehensive literature review about the age distribution of special vertigo diagnoses and also the data of the "German Vertigo Centre Munich" (n=500 consecutive patients). There, the incidence of dizziness syndromes in very elderly patients (> 80years) and young patients (<40years) were compared.

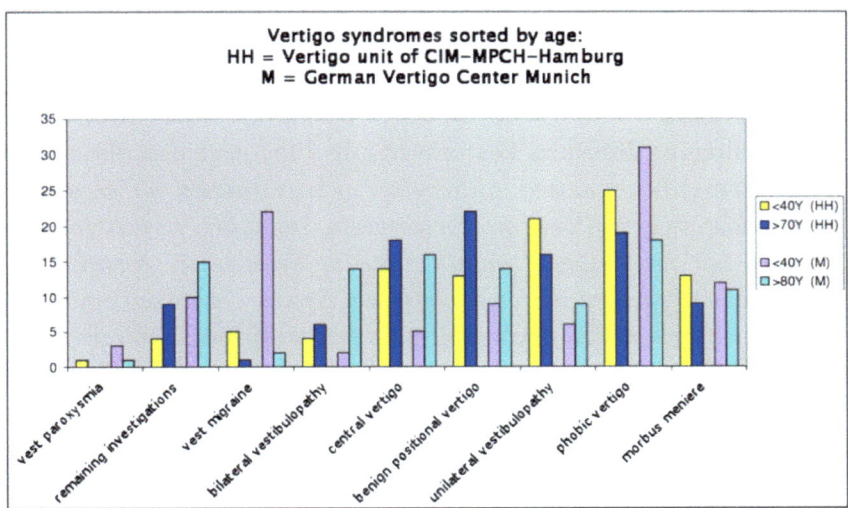

In Fig.2. *We have compared their results with our own findings from the University neurology clinic and the CIM-MPCH from the past 5 years (n = 562; "old"> 70years, "young" <40years).*

Mixed emotions and Anxiety

Many patients use the word dizziness to express in medical terms other feelings or disorders. Fear or verbally difficult to describe mixed emotions may be expressed in this way; such as *stunned horror, drowsiness, reduction of vigilance or concentration, instability in walking and grasping, but also feeling of emptiness during hypotension, hypoglycemic conditions, or hyperventilation phenomena.* Anxiety or mixed emotions that are difficult to describe are often expressed through "dizziness", a complaint like weakness. As a symptom of a general aid-searching with the doctor, "dizziness" is of a particularly good mixed significance. Complaints about dizziness provide therefore a special approach for patients who think that one should not go to the doctor for a general need for help, but must present him with a symptom: *Where there is no pain, there can be at least some dizziness.*

Time course of dizziness

The first diagnostic question therefore depends on the phenomenological classification of the complaints. That is, characteristics, timing, triggering conditions and accompanying symptoms of vertigo must be analyzed. If it is in the proper sense, vertigo is expressed mostly as a turning sensation, that the environment revolves around the patient, or the patient feels himself rotating in the environment. In the same way feelings of vertical uplift vertigo, or of being pulled into the ground are frequently reported. In terms of timing, we distinguish permanent vertigo, attacks of vertigo and seconds of vertigo. Quasi *permanent vertigo* reaches within minutes to hours a maximum and lasts several days. *Attacks of vertigo* occur randomly and may last between minutes and hours.

Finally, *seconds of vertigo* may occur during fast head movements or positional changes of the body. While in this case movement of the head or the whole body is important per se for triggering this *positional vertigo*, we differentiate *postural vertigo* that occurs in certain *body positions* and *body postures only*.

Dizziness – Functional Anatomy

With the question of the origin of vertigo arises the question of the anatomical substrate of vertigo. Because with characteristics and temporal course of a certain kind of vertigo, if well defined, we can draw conclusions about where this symptom originated. The primary organ of equilibrium or the vestibular organ consists of the two pairs of three semicircular canals that measure angular acceleration in the three spatial axes. Linear acceleration is measured by the also paired otoliths, in particularly gravity. This peripheral information is transferred to the vestibular nuclei of the brainstem, the phylogenetically oldest structure of our central nervous system, and in close connection with this to the cerebellum.

These signals are then passed through the pathways of the spinal cord and eventually to the limb muscles to control posture and movement coordination of the body. In the other direction, the complex equilibrium information is transmitted to the cerebral cortex through the thalamus, particularly to the parietal brain, and integrated with kinaesthetic information from other sensory organs: the visual system, the motion sensitivity of the joints and muscles of the extremities, and acoustic *motion impressions*. It is obvious that the symmetry and uniform integration of equilibrium messages may be disrupted at various points of these functional circuits.

Systematic and Time-defined Vertigo

In general one could say, the systematic and time-defined vertigo arises likely in the periphery i.e. in the area of the actual balance organ, the inner ear or at the transmission of information to the brain stem nuclei, the vestibular nerve. Secondarily, higher integration loci of bilaterally recorded equilibrium information leads to more complex phenomena of vertigo and dizziness. The idea of imbalance, of a sensory conflict or mismatch helps in understanding these phenomena. Thus, a disturbance of motion perception in the cervical spine and the neck muscles due to deficits of the vestibulospinal connections may result in positional vertigo; false spectacle prescriptions, latent squint or double vision in pareses of individual ocular muscles may lead to visual vertigo. In both cases, the mismatch of competing sensory perceptions results in vertigo.

Dizziness in a stricter sense

Dizziness in a stricter sense means a vertigo associated with feelings of displeasure, referred to disturbance of spatial orientation , or the perception of actually non-existent movement of the the environment or the body (turning/fluctuation). Vertigo corresponds to a disturbance of perception and is associated with disruption of gaze stabilization (nystagmus), disruption of posture control (postural instability) and of the autonomic nervous system with nausea / vomiting. A loss of orientation in space, is mostly characterized by neurovegetative signs and unpleasant feelings as: Nausea, sweating, blood pressure swings, anxiety, dysequilibrium of the sensory systems of reference: eye, balance, somatosensory perception in the space of reference. Initially, dizziness is often a complaint that is blurry described and not a clear symptom, syndrome or disease entity.

Clinical analysis of the ambiguous vertigo information

The usually ambiguous information provided by the patient who suffers from "Vertigo" has to be analyzed only by means of a careful history in conjunction with neuro-ophthalmological and neuro-otologic examination. These differentiate firstly a peripheral-vestibular from a centrally-vestibular form of vertigo. Additional apparative studies are of course necessary. Episodic vertigo with balance disorders usually indicates acute dysfunction of the vestibular system [peripheral or central] with a characteristic explanation of disturbed interaction of sensory systems: visual, vestibular, somatosensoric. In this respect vertigo sensu strictiori is always an indication of dysfunction of these multimodally connected systems. Physiologic vertigo may occur following being exposed to motion for a prolonged period such as when on a ship or simply following spinning with the eyes closed. Other causes may include toxin exposures such as to carbon monoxide, alcohol, or aspirin. Vertigo is a problem in a part of the vestibular system. Other causes of dizziness include presyncope, disequilibrium, and non-specific dizziness.

Vertigo – the most common type of dizziness: Frequent Diagnoses

With vertigo may be associated nausea, vomiting, sweating, or difficulties walking. It is typically worsened when the head is moved. The most common diseases that result in vertigo are benign paroxysmal positional vertigo, Ménière's disease, and labyrinthitis. Less common causes include stroke, brain tumors, brain injury, multiple sclerosis, and migraines.

Benign paroxysmal positional vertigo is more likely in someone who gets repeated episodes of vertigo with movement and is otherwise normal between these episodes. The episodes of vertigo should last less than one minute. The Dix-Hallpike test typically produces a period of rapid eye movements known as nystagmus in this condition. In Ménière's disease there is often ringing in the ears, hearing loss, and the attacks of vertigo last more than fifteen minutes. In labyrinthitis the onset of vertigo is sudden and the nystagmus occurs without movement. In this condition vertigo can last for days. More severe causes should also be considered. This is especially true if other problems such as weakness, headache, double vision, or numbness occur.

   Sudden vertigo attacks are not without danger, for example, if they occur while driving or lead to a fall. The fear associated therewith, like acrophobia, can become independent and lead to long-lasting symptoms: Phobic postural vertigo is particularly common as the sole cause, or as secondary cause of dizziness – but not vertigo sensu strictiori. In the second most frequent form of vertigo, the benign positional vertigo [BPV], that may follow attrition or light head concussions, is caused by broken small crystals of calcium carbonate (lime) in the inner ear that now float within the semicircular canals of the vestibular system: At each change of position they sink to the deepest point and the liquid is then accelerated in the semicircular canal: The patient experiences short, violent attacks of rotational vertigo. With a simple positioning maneuver, these lime particles are flooding out of the semicircular canals and so the symptoms are relieved in up to 90 %.

Also, unilateral or bilateral loss of the vestibular organs, inflammatory changes of the vestibular nerve as well as Meniere's disease always lead to vertigo. Less frequently but not less importantly, vertigo-migraine, neuro-degenerative diseases, and especially circulatory disorders of the brain stem or cerebellum must be seen by the neurologist: If dizziness/vertigo is accompanied by visual, speech, or movement disorders of the arms and legs, this is an emergency. A too high or too low blood pressure often leads to dizziness, lightheadedness, fainting or syncope.

Diagnostic Tests

Considerations in the neuro-ophthalmological / neuro-otologic examination. Recording of: spontaneous, gaze, fixational, position, or positional nystagmus. Signs of central vestibular disorders and/or other neurological symptoms/signs that point to a possibly central disorder. Subsequently, examination of the oculomotor and the vestibular system: Examination of the eye position / motility (velocity, acceleration, latency), incl. cover test. Smooth pursuit eye movements, and suppression of the vestibular ocular reflex during smooth head movements and the optokinetic reflex movements. Recording of fast eye movements (saccades) under various conditions. Clinical testing of peripheral vestibular functions and the vestibulo-ocular reflex (VOR) by rapid head rotation with/without fixation of a stationary point. Investigation under socalled Frenzel glasses. Standing with eyes closed (Romberg-Trial), blind walking on the spot (Unterberger Trial). Investigations of balance and in the oculomotor laboratory with infrared electro-oculographic, and electro-nystagmographic recordings, incl. calorisation, and rotational tests; click-evoked vestibular-neck-potentials, as well as vestibular-eye-muscle-potentials; neurosonology.

Dizziness of psychosomatic origin

Historical Context. Dizziness develops when the soul has to direct its attention to the ever faster collapsing conceptions, until they push themselves into each other and increasingly a chaotic state occurs, which is felt as a loss of balance. This idea was based on the observation of the symptoms of sick people and on self-observation, less on philosophical considerations. Writers and doctors --one example was the dissertation by Friedrich Schiller--provided the material for a new psychology, which was the expression of a discourse of self-awareness that took into account the other side of reason, the feelings, drives and passions. This discourse of self-awareness eventually led to Sigmund Freud's psychoanalysis.

Immanuel Kant[8], the most influential philosopher of the time, doubted the new philosophical medicine and suspected that the nature of the connection between body and thought could never be revealed. Kant criticized self-observation in particular, namely *"that the all too precise observation of oneself easily leads to madness if it is not already an expression of a mental illness. Whoever looks too deeply into his own abysses does not make a diagnosis, but only shows symptoms"*. The possibility of the experience to hold the things to be observed in the mind in order to bring them into a manageable order is not possible when observing uncalled thoughts and ideas that flow disorderly into consciousness. The order of thought always happens after the disorder of incoming thoughts, ideas, dreams, – and is replaced by vertigo and fear after the ever increasing disorder.

The perceptions must be logically connected to a whole of experience, so that we can speak of empirical knowledge as science. Kant: "Not observing but experimenting is the means to uncover nature and its forces." As it should turn out, observing and experimenting are not opposites but siblings. In 1820, when the Bohemian physiologist Jan

Evangelista Purkyně (see also Appendix) in his *"Beyträge zur näheren Kenntnis des Schwindels aus heautognostischen Daten"*[9] [meaning: autognostic, whz] operated with the terms dizziness and vertigo in the border region between physical and mental phenomena, this was for him just a classificatory differentiation. Vertigo thus became a psychophysical phenomenon that was exclusively attributable to material processes in the brain.

In modern context. Dizziness of psychosomatic origin is a non-systematic vertigo. It occurs rarely through a direct illness or injury of the vestibular system or its direct connections, but more often indirectly through sensory deficits of ocular, sensory or acoustic origin. Most frequently this diffuse, unsystematic dizziness will occur as the main symptom of general circulatory disorders, and therefore called *vascular insufficiency*. Often there are complaints about permanent vertigo, which lead to an intimate integration with psychological mechanisms. Focusing on the experience of vertigo can become a subjective expression of a painfully experienced age regression. It can also serve as a rationalizing explanation for a general failure of strength. Parkinson patients may develop dizziness and anxiety symptoms after repeated drops that may hamper their mobility more intensely than the primarily Parkinson induced movement disorder. The numerous older, mostly lonely patients who do not leave their home after a short fainting through a transient cerebral circulatory disturbance due to dizziness, demonstrate the close link between such forms of vertigo with anxiety, regression, and the threat of falling. In general, the first sign of this phenomenon vertigo is indeed associated with great anxiety; only secondarily, psychologically complicating factors may occur. Thus, vegetative reflexes -most commonly from the stomach and the heart- may cause dizziness and also a narrowing of consciousness. A typical example occurred at the time of the visit of US President George Bush in Tokyo 1990, when he collapsed at a banquet due to a gastrointestinal infection, which the television station CNN almost led to report his sudden death. The ruined stomach, bladder dyskinesias, solar plexus hits in boxing, digital anal examination and urethral bouguration were already described by Oppenheim[10] (1905) as vegetative causes triggering vertigo.

Psychosomatic and Psychogenic

Many doctors and laymen use the terms psychogenic and psychosomatic in a confused manner. In our context, this distinction is crucial: A certain vertigo is psychogenic if it acts solely on the internal sensation level. An organically caused vertigo could be influenced by psychological factors – which would be a vertigo of psychosomatic origin. *"I believe that everyone is capable of vertiginous feelings, i.e. the fact that one thinks intensively on the operation of some imbalance or of the memory images of vertigo. What is well known to a subject awakens in itself. This applies particularly in neurasthenic individuals, in which the fear of vertigo and the idea of vertigo can trigger this sensation readily"*[10] (Oppenheim 1905). Thus after a slight head injury vertigo often points to a psychological complication in the processing of the accident. Any accident, especially if one suffers a head injury is inevitably associated with a psychological trauma: The internal coherence and the fundamental safety of the individual feels under serious threat. Interestingly, posttraumatic neurotic reactions with persistent dizziness develop more frequently with light head traumas than with serious ones. This could be due to the fact that in severe injuries of the brain the actual accident disappears through the accidental memory lapse; in the light head trauma this is constantly mentally present as an anxiety source.

Phobic Vertigo

The frequent manifestation of purely psychogenic vertigo is called phobic vertigo. These patients suffer in specific situations only. Their fear of destruction corresponds to this specific quality of experience with its combination of dizziness and vertigo and its subjective stance and gait insecurity. They feel organically ill and believe their anxiety is caused by dizziness not vice versa. Typical triggers include sensory stimuli such as high bridges, stairs and car rides on narrow lanes; or social stress situations in supermarkets, restaurants or at meetings with the tendency to rapid conditioning and development of avoidance behaviour. Through an anxious introspection a mismatch is triggered between movement experience and its subjective internal copy, so that active body and head movements are experienced as passive accelerations or apparent movement. Their vertigo is explained accordingly: A cognitive dissonance in the perception of proportions is generated with this pre-existing anxious expectation. The resulting sense of vertigo triggers fearful panic, precisely because of this anxious expectation.

Johann Wolfgang Goethe applied a deconditioning therapy by frequent repetition of the anxiety-provoking experience, i.e. *the dissonance* between visual depth perception and sensory static near perception of the upright stand. The close connection between external stimulus conditions and the vertigo triggering sets generates this kind of vertigo. This explanation suggests that it is the result of a sequence of inconspicuous and in individual cases disturbed cognitive processing of vertiginous stimuli. Goethe[11] wrote about acrophobia in *Dichtung und Wahrheit* (poetry and truth). ... *"particularly frightened me a dizziness that always came over me when I looked down from a high altitude. Of these deficiencies I sought remedy in a highly efficient way, because I did not want to lose any time. After dinner at the Zapfenstreich* (zuck, last call) *I walked beside the drummers whose violent swirls and strokes were so strong that my heart could explode. I climbed alone to the highest peak of the Strassburg Münster tower and sat in the so-called neck under the head or the crown a quarter of an hour long; until I dared to step out into the open air, where you can stay on a disk that has a very small area, without being able to step, just standing, with the infinite country right there – however, the immediate vicinities and ornaments, the church and whatever one is seeing were hidden! It is quite as if you feel risen to a Mongolfiere* (hot air balloon) *into the air. Such things I repeated quite often with fear and anguish, until their impression was utterly indifferent."*

In the Alfred Hitchcock movie *Vertigo* James Stewart, playing the hero, faints while climbing a stepladder early on in the movie. He has to resign from the police force after an accident that causes him to develop both acrophobia and vertigo and throughout the movie the fear of heights and falling is repeatedly mentioned.

Phobia and Psychoanalysis

From a psychoanalytic perspective it should be added that the perception of certain situations could trigger fear. Since the experience of a large width or height may activate unconscious fantasy systems. This develops in the patient's field of action until she is so scared that *the foundation under her feet gets lost.* The loss of a stable external orientation through conflicting or unusual surrounding stimuli shows abruptly the lack of guidance in their own mental situation that may be threatened by overpowering conflicts of desires. Here the basic, primary mental process has neither a temporal structure nor a physical reality with a correct image of the structured nature of spatial relationships.

Fearful Dreams

The regression of dream experiences shows flight dreams, dreams of fear of falling, and other dreams in which the dreamer changes her location within the room not in accordance with the laws of physics, but because of her psychological needs; such that she might experience different spatial positions at the same time or spin through the space. In the dream, the space relationship is incorporated within the psychological needs according to the dream and a psychological signifier. Thus, the deep hole into which the dreamer crashes, could indicate the idea of a crash into a depressed mood. At the same time, it could symbolize a reversal into the contrary with the desire for a terrific rise. Kohut[12] noted that *"the narcissistic unmodified self pushes the ego to jump into the deep, to float through space or to fly. However, the real ego reacts with fear to those of his parts who wish to obey the life-threatening call."*

Incomprehensible and confusing emotions

Seemingly spontaneous psychogenic dizziness sensations arise in view of the individually incomprehensible, confusing emotions or inner perceptions that trigger anxiety. This is the classic vertigo complaint of the student in *Goethe's Faust* [13]:

"I will become by all this very silly, as if a mill would wheel within my the head ". As an anxiety equivalent the psychogenic dizziness sensation signals that the psychic equilibrium is threatened, destabilized or already decompensated. A vertigo signal indicates the fact that the synthetic function of the ego is disturbed. Vertigo may also serve to fend off a painful emotion – paradoxically for the subject often more tolerable – that may replace especially strong fear or feelings of guilt. The psychic economy draws here advantage from the circumstance that for the self the psychological relationship between the agonizing emotion and the underlying conflict is no longer visible. This creates a relief for the subject – if only apparently.

In addition to the replacement, there is also vertigo's function as coverage. So, vertigo may be used to cover hidden desires and may occur because of a prohibited or offensive relationship. We find a special proximity of dizziness with violent anger or deep shame of disgust in complaints of patients about permanent nausea or functional vomiting.

Regression: Fear and Psychogenic Vertigo

As a regressive phenomenon, psychogenic vertigo refers to the feeling of an impending loss of inner balance and thus to the time of transition from being hold and carried by the mother to the self-determined upright standing and running. In this perspective, the vertigo experience is the regressive revival of early child feelings with an anxiety-like experience while riding on roller coasters or similar driving devices that bring the balance system in flash: And this can be staged like a recalled image. Knowledge about the stability of the movement device is the basic requirement to enjoy the roaring ride. Vertigo occurs when the internal security and security-promoting object image is threatened. The analysis of vertigo experience thus pushes repeatedly on emotions or experiences that threaten the internal coherence of the subject in different ways. At the turn to the twentieth century, Freud[13] has described this situation: *"The vertigo of anxiety neurosis is neither vertigo, nor is it distinguished by individual planes and directions, and yet it belongs to the locomotor or coordinatory vertigo, nor as visual vertigo with eye muscle paralysis. It is a special discomfort accompanied by feelings of bottom surging; the legs sink, so that it is impossible to keep further upright, while the legs are leaden, tremble or buckle. This kind of vertigo never leads to falls."* As noted, complaints of vertigo are often found in depressive states, especially in neurotic depression. Here, the vertigo complaint can be the downright formation of the depressive content. Especially after object loss, it is the inner relationship framework through which the patient has structured his inner world, that is often under serious threat. The patient experiences a new freedom that *makes him dizzy*. A quote from the "*philosophy of fear*" by Søren Kierkegaard[14] concludes our considerations about "*the call of the void*":

"Fear can be compared with the experience of vertigo. The one whose eye suddenly looks down in to a yawning depth, will also become dizzy. But

what is the reason for this? It is as much his eye as the abyss; for what if he had not stared in to the abyss? So his fear is the dizziness of freedom, created by the mind that wants to set the synthesis! The freedom now looks down in to their possibility and grasps the finiteness to adhere to it. Through this vertigo freedom decreases and passes out."

Note on Purkinye.

Jan Evangelista **Purkinye** (1787-1869) ^{ref 4} *was born in Libochovice, Bohemia (now Czechoslovakia) and educated by Piarist monks. He studied philosophy at the University of Prague, was ordained a priest and became Father Salverius. In 1819, aged 32, he graduated in medicine. Purkinje, who had already made significant contributions to physiology, applied unsuccessfully for several University appoint-ments within the Austro-Hungarian Empire. Through friendship with Goethe he was appointed Professor of Physiology at Breslau University in 1823 against the opposition of the Faculty. In 1850 he was invited to the Chair of Physiology in Prague which he held until his death. His early work included the influence of the head position on the directional component of vertigo, and the maintenance of posture and equilibrium, culminating in Purkinje's Law of Vertigo. Purkinje explored aspects of vision and discovered in 1825 a phenomenon known as the Purkinje effect (as light intensity decreases, red objects are perceived to fade faster than blue objects). In 1837 he located the Purkinje cells in the cerebellar cortex, and two years later the Purkinje fibres lying beneath the endocardium. Purkinje also introduced the term protoplasm to describe the living embryonic material of the egg. He made original contributions to the histology of sweat glands, skin, bone, dental structures and was the first to discover the uniqueness of the human fingerprint.*

References

1. Lord Brain. Br Med J. 1963 ; 1(5333): 771–777
2. Jongkees LBW. Laryngoscope 1965; 79: 1473–1484
3. Marcus Herz. Versuch über den Schwindel". Felix Meiner Publishers Hamburg, Philosophische Bibliothek Bd.711, ed. by Bettina Stangneth, ISBN 978-3-7873-3447-6, 2019
4. Purkinje Jan Evangelista (1787-1869) in: LF Haas – *The maintenance of posture and equilibrium and Purkinje's Law of Vertigo.* J Neurol Neurosurg Psychiatry 1994; 57: 777
5. Stenger HH. *Schwindelanalyse.* European Archives of Oto-Rhino-Laryngology, 1959; 175, 545–549
6. Kestenbaum P and P Vogel, ref. in: Paul Enoksson, *Optokinetic nystagmus in brain lesions,* Acta Ophthlmologica 1956; 3: 163 – 184
7. Jahn K et al. Review . Deutsches Aerzteblatt 2015; 112: 387-93
8. Kant I. *Prolegomena to any future metaphysics.* Bobbs-Merrill Company, Inc., New York 1949. Orig.: Prolegomena zu einer jeden künftigen Metaphysik, die als Wissenschaft wird auftreten können. Frankfurt & Leipzig 1794.
9. Purkinje JE: *Beyträge zur näheren Kenntnis des Schwindels aus heautognostischen Daten.* In: *Medicinische Jahrbücher des k. k. österreichischen Staates.* Wien 1820 a, VI. II. Stück, S. 79–125.
10. Oppenheim H. *Die traumatischen Neurosen* (1889) and *Lehrbuch der Nervenkrankheiten* (7th ed.)1923
11. Goethe JW. *Dichtung und Wahrheit.* Publ. Cotta, Stuttgart und Tuebingen 1812
12. Kohut H. *The Analysis of the Self. A Systematic Approach to the Psychoanalytic Treatment of Narcissistic Personality Disorders.* International Universities Press, New York 1971
13. Goethe JW.. *Faust I.* Publ. Cotta Stuttgart und Tuebingen 1808
14. Quinodoz Jean-Michel. *Reading Freud. A Chronological Exploration of Freud's Writings.* Routledge, New Library of Psychoanalysis

Teaching Series, 2006, Paperback No. 2005-07-14 .Faust I, Vers 1946 f. / Schüler". Aus: Johann Wolfgang von Goethe, Dramen, Faust. Eine Tragödie (1808)

15. Kierkegaard S, *Der Begriff Angst*. Kopenhagen 1844
16. A clinical description and therapeutic advice concerning vertigo in English and German can be found here: http://www.schwin-del-sprechstunde-hamburg.de/en/en-startpage/

Cover: Klaus Kumrow, O.T., Aquarell, 1986
